GW01017949

Forestry First Aid

Forestry First Aid is published by: **Nuco Training Ltd**

INTRODUCTION TO FORESTRY FIRST AID

It is recommended that anyone working in forestry or agricultural operations should undertake additional first aid training delivered with a forestry context. This is due to the nature of the work and the increased risk of injury or illness in remote environments.

People willing to undertake the Forestry First Aid course must hold (or be working towards) an Emergency First Aid at Work or First Aid at Work qualification prior to attending.

By completing the Forestry First Aid programme, you will gain the knowledge and skills required to deal with a range of topics which extend beyond that of a workplace first aid course.

Forestry First Aid training should be repeated every 3-years in line with your First Aid at Work or Emergency First Aid at Work qualification. Annual refresher training is also advised to keep your knowledge and skills up-to-date.

THE HEALTH AND SAFETY (FIRST AID) REGULATIONS 1981
(1982 IN NORTHERN IRELAND)

The Health and Safety (First Aid) Regulations 1981 require employers to provide adequate and appropriate equipment, facilities and personnel to ensure their employees receive immediate attention if they are injured or taken ill at work.

The term 'at work' encompasses lone working, travelling and when you are on site temporarily to complete a task. The regulations also apply to self-employed personnel.

You should liaise with management and other First Aiders to ensure:

- **There is an adequate number of First Aiders and Emergency First Aiders in place**
- **Appropriate equipment, kits and facilities are available in suitable locations across the site**
- **A system is in place to manage medical emergencies and to report incidents and accidents**

It is vital that an assessment of first aid needs is conducted to ensure the correct level of provision is made. This will be covered in section 2 of this manual.

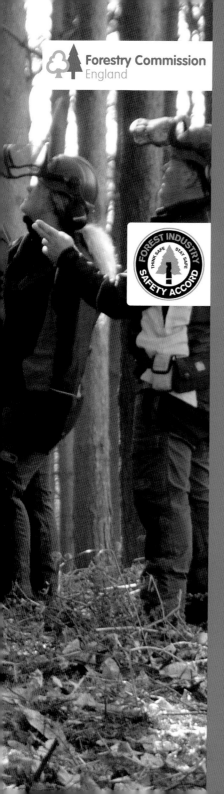

FORESTRY COMMISSION FIRST AID AT WORK POLICY

In addition to complying with national legislation, anyone wishing to work on Forestry Commission (FC) land should follow the Forestry Commission First Aid at Work policy.

This policy document sets out the approach to first aid provision in a forestry context. It shows the minimum standards for those working on Forestry Commission managed land, and includes example scenarios of what to record in your assessment of first aid needs.

For more information, please visit: **www.forestryengland.uk/article/first-aid-policy**

FISA SAFETY GUIDE 802 EMERGENCY PLANNING

It is advised that the Forestry Commission First Aid at Work policy should be followed in conjunction with the 'FISA802 *(Emergency Planning)'* guidance leaflet.

This guidance leaflet is produced by the Forest Industry Safety Accord (FISA) who set out the industries commitment to raising health, safety and welfare standards in the workplace.

The purpose of this guidance is to help minimise the time taken for the emergency services to reach you and recommend ways to minimise the risks to operators if there is an emergency. It also highlights the need to include environmental and other types of emergency within the planning process.

For more information, please visit: **www.ukfisa.com/safety-information/safety-library/fisa-safety-guides**

ASSESSMENT OF FIRST AID NEEDS

To determine the level of first aid equipment, facilities and personnel required in the workplace, you should consider the following factors:

- **The nature of the work and the hazards and risks involved**
- **History of accidents and illnesses and the resulting consequences**
- **Distribution of the workforce, shift times and work patterns**
- **Remoteness of sites, lone workers and travelling arrangements**
- **Absenteeism of First Aiders, annual leave and provision for non-employees**

Planning for an emergency in advance can often be over-looked when it comes down to assessing your first aid needs, although it is one of the most important elements of Forestry First Aid.

The overall aim of emergency planning is to ensure your casualty receives medical assistance as soon as possible following an incident.

Many forestry and agricultural sites are distant from urban areas and you may be caring for your casualty for an extended period of time. The emergency services may need assistance from the local mountain rescue team if access and egress is going to cause a problem reaching the casualty.

You can have all the necessary skills and equipment to administer first aid, but when you are on your own without any procedures to follow, lives can be put at risk.

GENERAL SAFETY MEASURES TO ENSURE THE HEALTH AND SAFETY OF THE WORKFORCE

If it is possible, avoid working alone. Arrangements should be made for someone to check on you at regular intervals. The greater the risk, the more frequent the checks should be. As a minimum, always inform your point of contact when you start and finish work.

If you are part of a team distributed across a large area, you should arrange to meet up at regular intervals throughout the day.

Each team member should carry a personal first aid kit (or travel kit) in addition to the workplace first aid kits, which should be kept at key locations across the site.

The responsible person should carry out the assessment of first aid needs to determine the equipment, facilities and personnel required to ensure there is immediate assistance available to workers who suffer illness or injury.

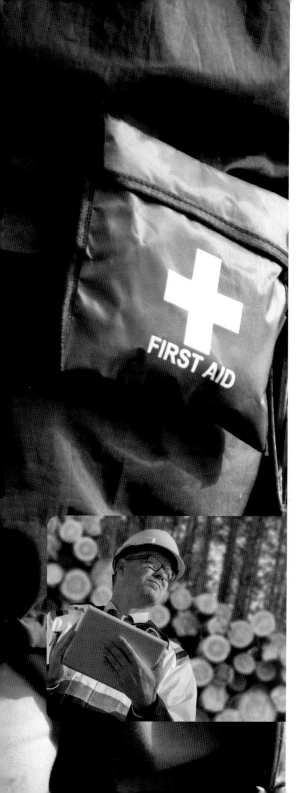

PLANNING FOR AN EMERGENCY

For emergency procedures to work well, it is vital that all operators and managers are aware of the procedures and have had the opportunity to test them.

Factors to consider when planning for an emergency can include:

- Identifying the personnel and equipment that needs to be on site and on person in case of an emergency
- Identifying significant hazards and implementing suitable control measures
- Anticipating difficulties that may exist reaching the casualty; the emergency services will need to access the site without delay
- Checking mobile phone reception and introducing alternative methods of communication such as radio transceivers
- If chemicals are to be used, you must ensure that a risk assessment has been carried out and you have a plan in place in case of spillages (consider; emergency contacts, emergency spill kits, storage, PPE etc)
- Identification of mains services (overhead and underground) and the relevant emergency contact details for each service
- The emergency services may dispatch a helicopter to your location if it is necessary. You should include this in your emergency plans and consider a suitable area for landing

Emergency procedures should be tested, evaluated, documented and revised as necessary.

ACTION IN AN EMERGENCY

Emergency procedures will vary, but the overall aims of administering first aid and summoning professional medical assistance will be similar throughout the industry.

- If there is an emergency, make sure the area is safe for you, the casualty and anyone in the vicinity
- Look out for hazards (above, below and around) such as high-voltage electricity cables and dangerous machinery. Do not put yourself in danger
- Administer first aid to the casualty following the primary survey (DR<C>ABC) – see page 9
- Contact the emergency services and explain clearly what has happened. Stay on the line so that the operator can provide advice and support whilst waiting for professional help to arrive

WHEN HELP IS MORE THAN 30 MINUTES AWAY

If it is possible, insulate your casualty from the ground before placing them in the recovery position. Provide a form of shelter and keep them warm by covering their body using a foil blanket or spare clothing.

If they have been kept in the recovery position for more than 30 minutes, turn them to the opposite side to relieve pressure on the lower arm. You will need to turn the casualty every 30 minutes until professional help arrives on scene.

You should also monitor the casualty's vital signs at regular intervals which will help you identify problems and indicate any changes to their condition.

Vital signs are measurements of the body's most basic functions which include their verbal response, breathing, pulse, skin colour and their body temperature.

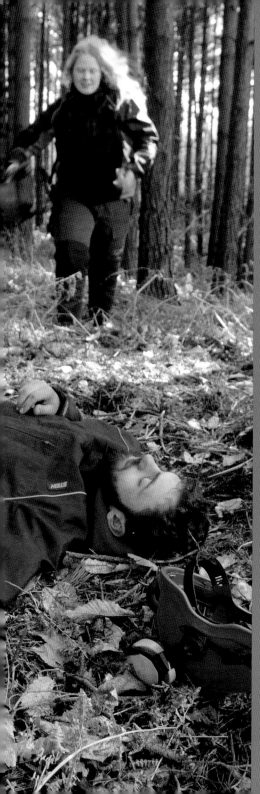

CONTACTING THE EMERGENCY SERVICES

The emergency services can be contacted by dialling 999/112. The operator will ask a series of questions so the emergency services vehicle can reach you as quickly as possible.

The emergency services operator may ask you for:

- **Your location**
- **Your name and contact details**
- **What has happened and when?**
- **Casualty's age, gender and known medical history**
- **Nature and extent of injuries or illness (if known)**
  - **Is the casualty responsive?**
  - **Are they breathing normally?**
  - **Is there severe bleeding?**
  - **Are they experiencing chest pain?**
  - **What treatment has already been given?**
- **How close can the emergency services vehicle get to the area?**
- **Are there any significant hazards the rescue services need to be aware of?**

MOUNTAIN RESCUE

It may prove challenging for an ambulance to reach you when you are in a remote setting. You may need help from the local mountain rescue team who will have all the necessary equipment and supplies to assist you. Depending on the situation, the 999 telephone operator may be able to make the arrangements for you.

The procedure for calling mountain rescue:

- **Dial 999/112**
- **Request "THE POLICE"**
- **Ask for "MOUNTAIN RESCUE"**

Mountain rescue teams work across mountain and moorland areas to carry out rescues in difficult-to-access areas. Each rescue team is a charity in their own right and all members are volunteers.

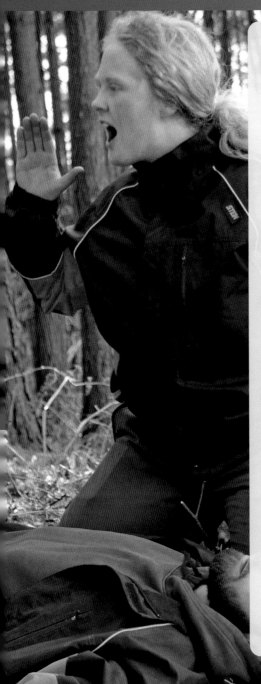

OTHER METHODS FOR SUMMONING ASSISTANCE

Shouting

Shouting for "HELP" loudly and clearly may alert passers-by that you need assistance. This can help with both incident management and summoning further help.

International Distress Signal

The International Distress Signal can be recognised by either 6 short blasts of a whistle or 6 flashes of a light repeated every minute. This should be continued even if someone is replying, commonly with 3 blasts or 3 flashes every minute.

SOS Morse Code

Although similar, Morse Code differs to the International Distress Signal and can be recognised by a number of different means, i.e. beeps on a radio, blasts of a whistle, flashes of a light, etc. It follows the same pattern: 3 short, 3 long, 3 short and repeat. The pattern is repeated every minute even if someone is replying, commonly with just 3 beeps, blasts or flashes.

Send a text

Sending a text requires much less signal strength compared to making a phone call. The phone will keep trying to send the text for a short period of time, meaning there is a greater chance of the message getting through if you are moving or in an area of changeable reception.

EMERGENCYSMS SERVICE

In the UK, EmergencySMS is a simple and innovative system that was designed to aid people who have a hearing or speech impairment to text the emergency services. It should be noted that a mobile phone must be registered with this service to use it.

To register:

Text "register" to 999. Read the reply text fully and once you reply with a "YES" your phone will be registered.

PRIMARY SURVEY

For any first aid incident, you will have learned in your first aid training about DR ABC. For a catastrophic bleed, the priorities of the primary survey now changes to:

D   **Check for dangers**

R   **Response**

C   **Catastrophic bleed identified**
This is now your priority. Summon professional medical help immediately and control the bleeding.

A   **Airway**

B   **Breathing**

C   **CPR / circulation**

Time is of the essence to control the bleeding as quickly and as effectively as you can and to treat the casualty for hypovolaemic shock *(hypovolaemia)*, which occurs when there is a decrease in blood volume or bodily fluid, which can be fatal.

FIRST AID GUIDELINES

There is very little literature comparing different bleeding control strategies commonly employed by First Aiders. The best control method for bleeding is to apply direct pressure to the wound where possible.

There is no published evidence for the effective use of proximal pressure points to control bleeding. In addition, do not try to control major external bleeding by the elevation of an extremity.

Where bleeding cannot be controlled by direct pressure, it may be possible to control bleeding by the use of a haemostatic dressing, or a tourniquet.

To summarise the first aid guidelines for catastrophic bleeding:

- **Do apply direct pressure to the wound**
- **Do use a haemostatic dressing or tourniquet**
- **Do not apply indirect pressure to proximal pressure points**
- **Do not elevate an extremity**

FIRST AID KITS

Where it is identified that there is a risk of catastrophic bleed injuries, as with the use of chainsaws, a specialist haemorrhage kit is advised, which should contain a minimum of:

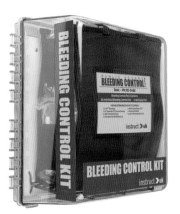

- **2 x Gloves**
- **4 x Pressure bandages**
- **2 x Haemostatic dressings**
- **4 x Tourniquets**
- **1 x Medical grade scissors**
- **1 x Marker pen**

This specialised kit would be in addition to your standard workplace first aid kit.

The view of the HSE is that the inclusion of these items is based on your assessment of first aid needs. Where your assessment has identified a requirement for tourniquets and/or haemostatic dressings, you should make sure:

- **Your haemostatic dressings are always in date**
- **Workplace First Aiders are trained by a competent provider**

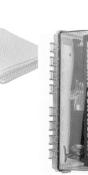

HYPOVOLAEMIA

Hypovolaemia is a decrease in the volume of blood in your body, which can be due to blood loss, or loss of body fluids. Blood loss can result from external injuries, internal bleeding, or certain obstetric emergencies in childbirth.

Diarrhoea and vomiting are common causes of body fluid loss. Fluid can also be lost as a result of large burns, excessive perspiration or diuretics (increased production of urine). Inadequate fluid intake can also cause hypovolaemia.

HYPOVOLAEMIC SHOCK (ALSO KNOWN AS HAEMORRHAGIC SHOCK)

Blood makes up about 7% of our body weight and an average adult has approximately 5 litres of blood in their body.

Effects of blood loss:

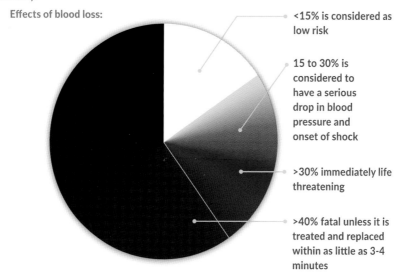

- <15% is considered as low risk

- 15 to 30% is considered to have a serious drop in blood pressure and onset of shock

- >30% immediately life threatening

- >40% fatal unless it is treated and replaced within as little as 3-4 minutes

This severe fluid loss makes it impossible for the heart to pump a sufficient amount of blood to the body and can lead to organ failure. This condition requires immediate emergency medical attention.

Symptoms of hypovolaemic shock may include:

- Catastrophic bleeding
- Anxiety
- Clammy skin
- Cold
- Confusion
- Decreased or absent urine output
- Paleness
- Rapid breathing and heart rate
- Sweating
- Weakness
- Unresponsiveness

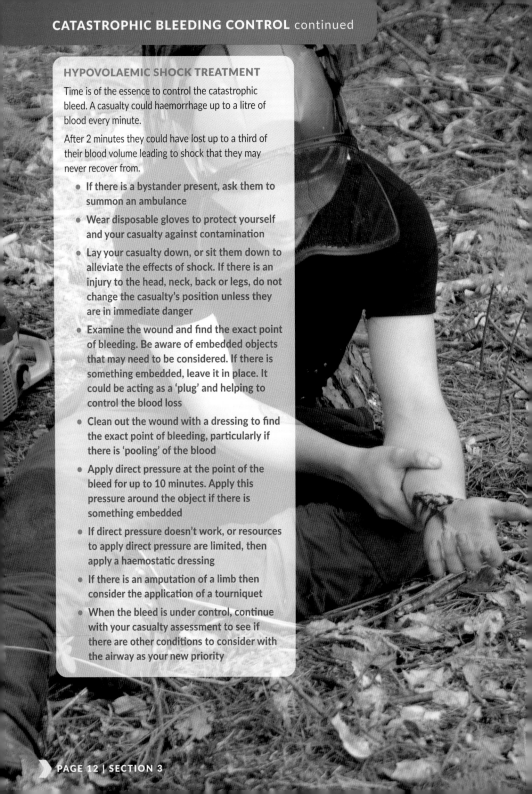

HYPOVOLAEMIC SHOCK TREATMENT

Time is of the essence to control the catastrophic bleed. A casualty could haemorrhage up to a litre of blood every minute.

After 2 minutes they could have lost up to a third of their blood volume leading to shock that they may never recover from.

- If there is a bystander present, ask them to summon an ambulance

- Wear disposable gloves to protect yourself and your casualty against contamination

- Lay your casualty down, or sit them down to alleviate the effects of shock. If there is an injury to the head, neck, back or legs, do not change the casualty's position unless they are in immediate danger

- Examine the wound and find the exact point of bleeding. Be aware of embedded objects that may need to be considered. If there is something embedded, leave it in place. It could be acting as a 'plug' and helping to control the blood loss

- Clean out the wound with a dressing to find the exact point of bleeding, particularly if there is 'pooling' of the blood

- Apply direct pressure at the point of the bleed for up to 10 minutes. Apply this pressure around the object if there is something embedded

- If direct pressure doesn't work, or resources to apply direct pressure are limited, then apply a haemostatic dressing

- If there is an amputation of a limb then consider the application of a tourniquet

- When the bleed is under control, continue with your casualty assessment to see if there are other conditions to consider with the airway as your new priority

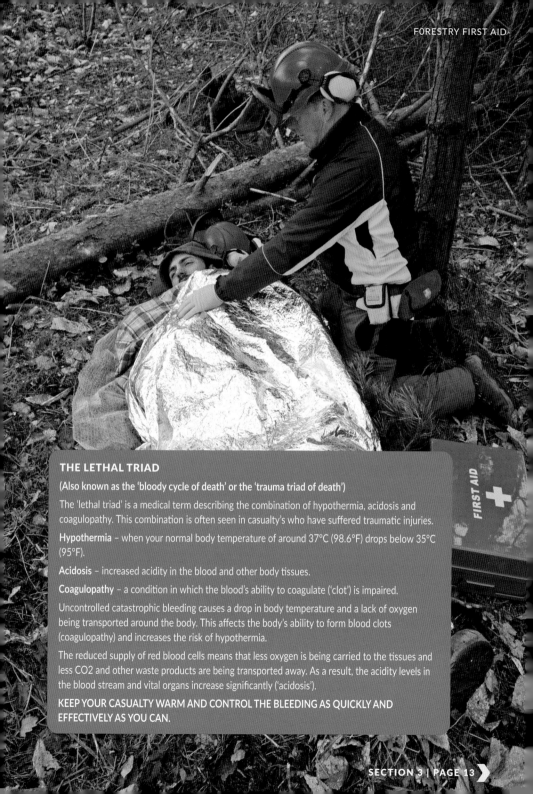

THE LETHAL TRIAD

(Also known as the 'bloody cycle of death' or the 'trauma triad of death')

The 'lethal triad' is a medical term describing the combination of hypothermia, acidosis and coagulopathy. This combination is often seen in casualty's who have suffered traumatic injuries.

Hypothermia – when your normal body temperature of around 37°C (98.6°F) drops below 35°C (95°F).

Acidosis – increased acidity in the blood and other body tissues.

Coagulopathy – a condition in which the blood's ability to coagulate ('clot') is impaired.

Uncontrolled catastrophic bleeding causes a drop in body temperature and a lack of oxygen being transported around the body. This affects the body's ability to form blood clots (coagulopathy) and increases the risk of hypothermia.

The reduced supply of red blood cells means that less oxygen is being carried to the tissues and less CO_2 and other waste products are being transported away. As a result, the acidity levels in the blood stream and vital organs increase significantly ('acidosis').

KEEP YOUR CASUALTY WARM AND CONTROL THE BLEEDING AS QUICKLY AND EFFECTIVELY AS YOU CAN.

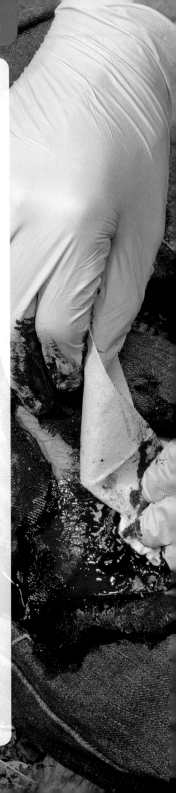

IMPROVISED TREATMENT

Treatment if you have no tourniquet or haemostatic dressing:

- If there is a bystander present, ask them to summon an ambulance
- Wear disposable gloves to protect yourself and the casualty against contamination
- Lay your casualty down, or sit them down to alleviate the effects of shock
- Examine the wound and find the exact point of bleeding. Be aware of embedded objects that may need to be considered. If there is something embedded, leave it in place. It could be acting as a 'plug' and helping to control the blood loss
- Clean out the wound with a dressing to find the exact point of bleeding, particularly if there is 'pooling' of the blood
- Apply direct pressure at the point of the bleed. Apply this pressure at the point of the bleed for up to 10 minutes. Apply this pressure around the object if there is something embedded
- Pack the wound with unfolded sterile dressings. Use as many as it takes to pack the wound
- Apply direct pressure on this packing
- Secure this packing with a sterile dressing, triangular bandage or similar item
- If blood seeps through this dressing, remove it and apply a new one

TOURNIQUET OR HAEMOSTATIC DRESSING?

There is no golden rule on whether a tourniquet should be used first opposed to a haemostatic dressing. However the site of injury, what you have available and the environment could be deciding factors.

You should NOT use a tourniquet on:

- The head
- The abdomen
- The neck
- The shoulders
- The groin

You should not pack the following wounds with haemostatic dressings:

- Open head injury
- Open chest injury

WHAT DOES HAEMOSTATIC MEAN?

Haemo: Blood

Static: At rest

HAEMOSTATIC DRESSINGS

A haemostatic dressing is a medical dressing used to control blood loss by accelerating the clotting process. The dressing is impregnated with a special agent that when it makes contact with a fluid (blood in this instance), it creates a gel around the point of where the blood is being lost which in essence acts as the clot, or pseudo clot.

This special agent also comes in a granular and powder form. The granular form is a very useful substitute for the haemostatic dressing, particularly for the smaller deeper wounds such as a gunshot or stabbing wound where a dressing cannot be easily applied.

There are many haemostatic dressings and agents on the market and they all have their own unique features. For the purposes of this publication, we will focus on Celox™ which is a well-known brand offering a variety of haemostatic products.

HOW CELOX™ PRODUCTS WORK

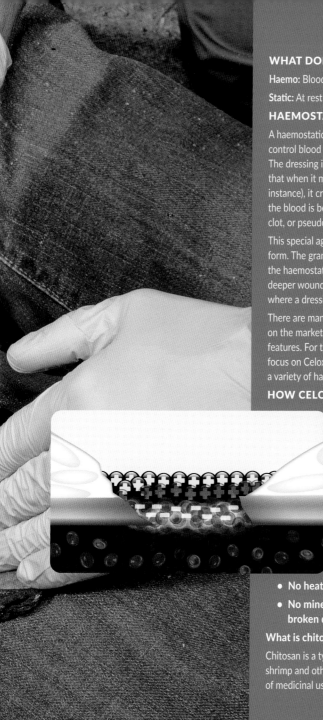

- Celox™ products contain chitosan, which absorbs fluid, swells and forms a gel substance to stop the bleeding
- Celox™ electrostatically attracts red blood cells and forms a gel-like plug
- Celox™ does not rely on the body's own clotting mechanism
- No heat generated
- No minerals. Residual chitosan is naturally broken down and excreted by the body

What is chitosan?

Chitosan is a type of sugar found in the shells of shrimp and other sea crustaceans. It has a wide range of medicinal uses, including haemorrhage control.

CELOX™ RAPID GAUZE

Celox™ RAPID gauze is a non-woven gauze, laminated with the proven Celox™ granules and individually sterile packed in a ruggedized pouch with tear notches for fast opening.

It is available in a compressed 5 foot Z-folded format and also as a 10 foot roll. The z-folded pack is ideal for the medic or vehicle kit, as it takes up less space.

Pack the gauze directly on to the bleeding source and hold pressure for three minutes to stop life-threatening bleeding from arterial injuries, gunshot wounds, road traffic accidents and other severe injuries.

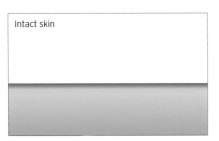

Intact skin

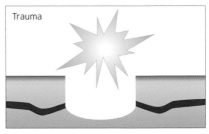

Trauma

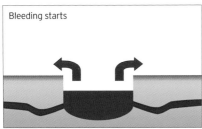

Bleeding starts

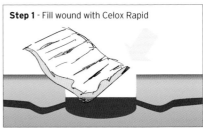

Step 1 - Fill wound with Celox Rapid

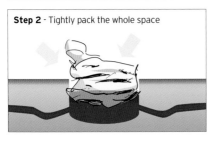

Step 2 - Tightly pack the whole space

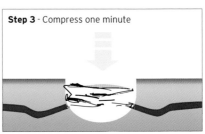

Step 3 - Compress one minute

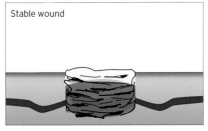

Stable wound

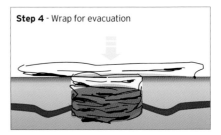

Step 4 - Wrap for evacuation

CELOX™-A HAEMOSTAT APPLICATOR

Penetrating injuries such as blast or knife wounds are very difficult to treat and are often lethal. It is vital to stop bleeding quickly.

Celox™-A is a unique haemostat applicator delivery system pre-packed with Celox™ granules and designed to get through a small entry wound, directly to the bleeding site in just a few seconds. Simple to use, it is the fastest and most effective haemostat applicator available.

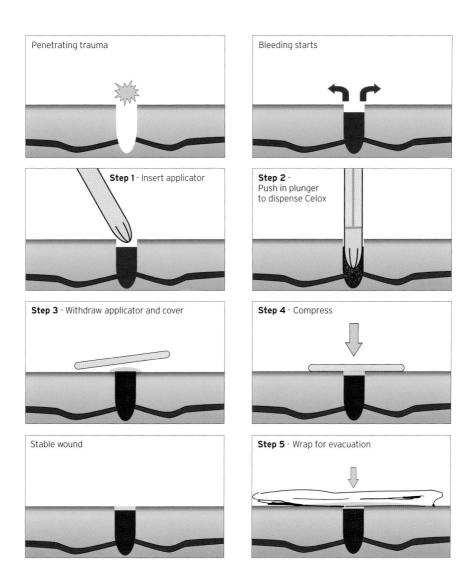

Penetrating trauma

Bleeding starts

Step 1 - Insert applicator

Step 2 - Push in plunger to dispense Celox

Step 3 - Withdraw applicator and cover

Step 4 - Compress

Stable wound

Step 5 - Wrap for evacuation

CELOX™ HAEMOSTATIC GRANULES

When mixed with blood, Celox™ forms a robust plug stopping bleeding in 5 minutes. It works independently of the body's normal clotting processes. Celox's™ clotting ability has been proven to work in the cold (hypothermia), or in the presence of common anti-coagulants such as Warfarin.
It generates no heat and will not burn the casualty or those offering the treatment.

In tests by the US Office of Naval Research, Celox™ was the only product to give 100% survival.
It gave a strong stable MAP (mean arterial blood pressure) and was also the only product to give robust clotting with no re-bleeding. Celox's™ safety has been tested to the intense class 3 CE mark standards.

Intact skin

Trauma

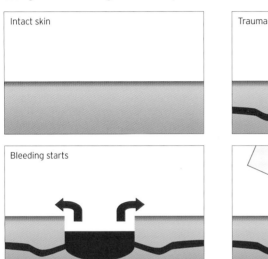

Bleeding starts

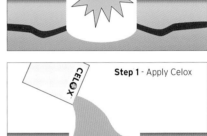

Step 1 - Apply Celox

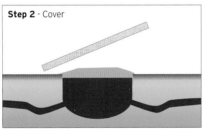

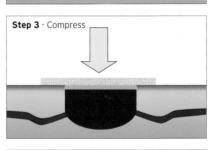

Step 2 - Cover

Step 3 - Compress

Stable wound

Step 4 - Wrap for evacuation

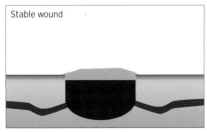

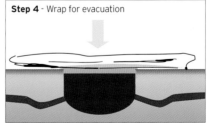

WHAT IS A TOURNIQUET?

A tourniquet is a device used to temporarily control arterial and venous blood flow to a portion of an extremity for a period of time. There are many tourniquets on the market and they all have their unique features and benefits.

- **A windlass is part of a tourniquet that is twisted to tighten it and is then locked or tied in place to secure the tourniquet when pressure is applied**
- **A tourniquet should be a minimum of 1.5 inches wide and this is particularly important if you have to improvise and make your own**
- **Unpack the manufactured tourniquet and have it ready to use**
- **Apply directly to the skin and not clothing**
- **Make sure you write the time of application on the tourniquet. Most manufactured ones will have an area designated for this**

TOURNIQUET PLACEMENT

It is advised that in emergency care practice, any necessary tourniquet should be applied as distally as possible above the wound on the same bone structure, to preserve the maximum amount of salvageable tissue.

Where access to the limb is limited, the tourniquet may need to be placed more proximally up the limb. In these cases, a review of the first placement should be considered with a view to re-apply the tourniquet closer to the wound, prior to releasing the initial, higher placed tourniquet. This is to make sure that haemorrhage control is maintained.

In blast injury (ragged wounds), large circumference limbs and situations where treatment is being applied early (the patient's blood pressure is high) it may be necessary to apply 2 tourniquets. The second tourniquet should be applied above the first. (see page 20)

It is important not to go too close to the knee joint as the femoral condyles offer some protection to the artery from the tourniquet as it passes between them.

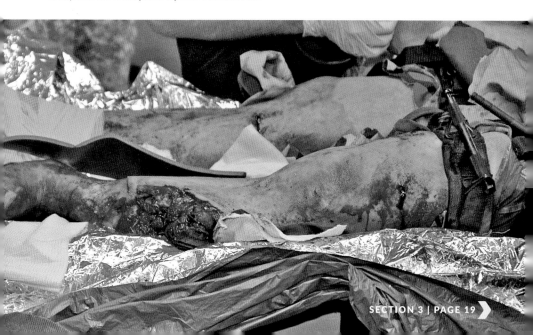

PLACE THE TOURNIQUET APPROXIMATELY TWO INCHES ABOVE THE POINT OF BLEEDING ON THE SAME BONE STRUCTURE.

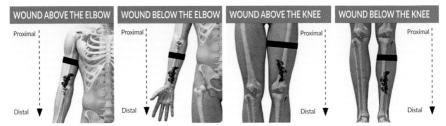

WOUND ABOVE THE ELBOW	WOUND BELOW THE ELBOW	WOUND ABOVE THE KNEE	WOUND BELOW THE KNEE
Proximal ... Distal ▼	Proximal ... Distal ▼	Proximal ... Distal ▼	Proximal ... Distal ▼

PLACEMENT OF 2 TOURNIQUETS

If the wound is to a distal part of the limb and the first tourniquet does not control the bleeding sufficiently, then consideration should be given to the application of a second tourniquet above the first.

If space is restricted to apply the second tourniquet directly above the first, it can be applied above the elbow/knee joint on the single bone structure.

Your aim is to stop the bleeding and preserve as much of the body tissue as possible.

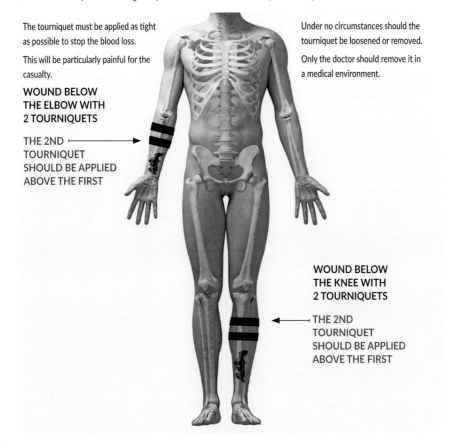

The tourniquet must be applied as tight as possible to stop the blood loss.

This will be particularly painful for the casualty.

WOUND BELOW THE ELBOW WITH 2 TOURNIQUETS

THE 2ND TOURNIQUET SHOULD BE APPLIED ABOVE THE FIRST

Under no circumstances should the tourniquet be loosened or removed.

Only the doctor should remove it in a medical environment.

WOUND BELOW THE KNEE WITH 2 TOURNIQUETS

THE 2ND TOURNIQUET SHOULD BE APPLIED ABOVE THE FIRST

WHAT ARE THE RISKS ASSOCIATED WITH A TOURNIQUET?

Loss of a limb

There is a general feeling throughout the first aid world that the application of a tourniquet will ultimately lead to a loss of limb.

The general medical consensus is that a tourniquet can be left on for up to 2 hours with little risk to muscle damage. The risk becomes much greater beyond this period and the likelihood of an amputation will almost be the case for up to 6 hours.

Remember that our aim in first aid is to preserve life and to prevent the injury from worsening. By stopping the bleeding, it may well keep your casualty alive.

The potential for a loss of a limb is outweighed by the potential for loss of life.

Not tight enough

Tourniquets only work if they are tight enough to stop arterial blood flow. Arterial blood is under significantly more pressure than venous blood, and it takes more pressure to stop it. Tourniquets should not be too narrow or they will cut into the skin as pressure is applied. The wider the tourniquet, the more pressure that is required to stop blood flow.

Generally speaking, for best results, tourniquets should be a minimum of 1.5 inches wide. Tourniquets on the leg will need to be narrower than those on the arm, due to the increased pressure necessary to stop the blood flow in the leg.

Risk of losing a limb

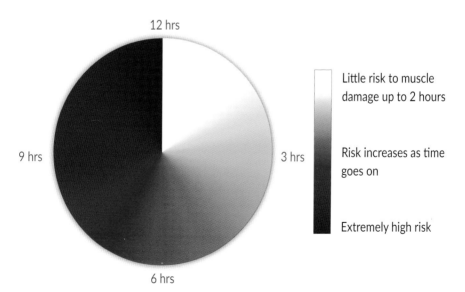

TOURNIQUET IMPROVISATION

Where a manufactured tourniquet is not available, an improvised one can be equally effective. It is important to achieve the right width of 1.5 inches, so a broad-fold bandage such as a triangular bandage would be an ideal resource. This should be folded to create a 1.5 inch wide strap and then tied off 5cms (2 inches) above the wound or joint.

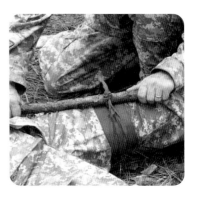

Do not use stretchy materials to make a tourniquet.

You can also improvise a windlass. Use a metal object such as a spoon that can be used to twist the tourniquet to the correct tightness and then tie the tourniquet off.

THE STEPWISE APPROACH IN DEALING WITH A CATASTROPHIC BLEED

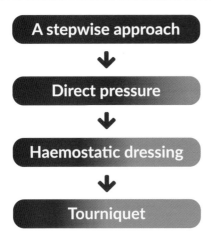

CASUALTY HANDOVER

A trusted structure for medical professionals in any casualty handover that is worth remembering and adopting is:

- **A**   Age and other patient details
- **T**   Time of incident
- **M**   Mechanism
- **I**   Injuries sustained
- **S**   Signs
- **T**   Treatment and trends

This structure enables all members involved in the patient care, both in hospital receiving teams and those delivering the patient to that care, to work in an expected and structured fashion with a dependable format.

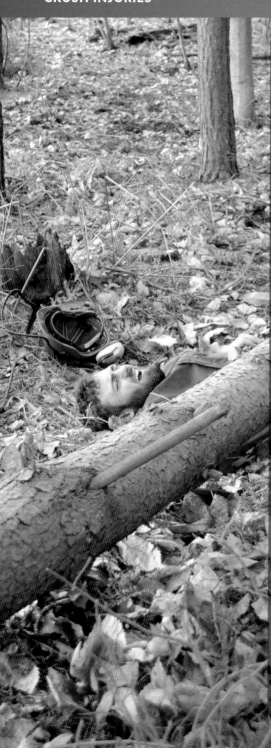

CRUSH INJURIES

A crush injury is a direct injury resulting from a crush where a body part has been subjected to a high degree of force or pressure, usually when a body part is squeezed between two objects.

Crush injuries can affect the flow of blood to the limb that is being crushed, restricting fresh oxygen reaching the limb and a build up of waste products will start to accumulate.

When the waste products reach a toxic level and the limb is released from the crush, these toxins will enter the circulatory system which can cause 'crush syndrome'.

Due to the risk of crush syndrome, the current recommendation for First Aiders is to not release the casualty who has been trapped for more than 15 minutes.

For major crush injuries, symptoms may include:

- **Severe pain**
- **Catastrophic bleeding**
- **Limb deformity**
- **Internal injuries**
- **Paresthesia** (tingling sensations)
- **Numbness**
- **Fractures**
- **Bruising**

CRUSH SYNDROME

The severe systemic manifestation of muscle cell damage and the restriction of blood flow, resulting from a body part being crushed by an object for a prolonged period of time.

When the pressure is released from the crushed limb, large quantities of metabolites (such as potassium, phosphate and urate) will leak into the circulatory system, be pumped to our vital organs and cause serious health complications.

Crush syndrome is also known as Bywaters' syndrome.

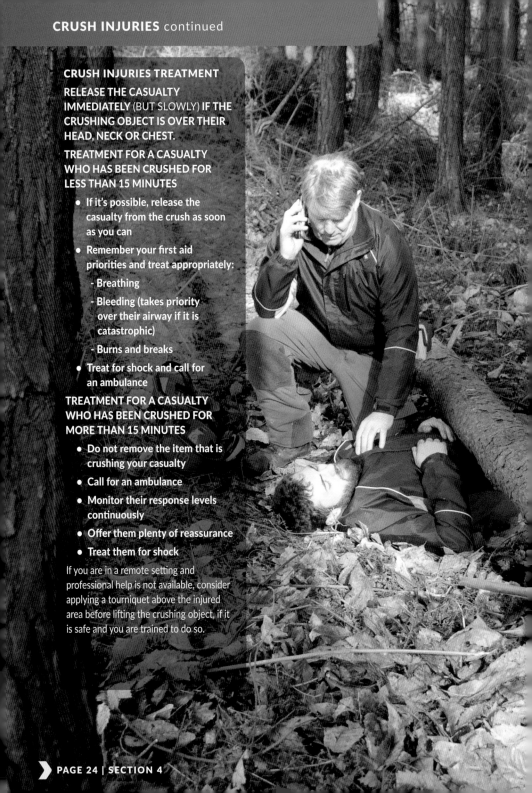

CRUSH INJURIES TREATMENT

RELEASE THE CASUALTY IMMEDIATELY (BUT SLOWLY) **IF THE CRUSHING OBJECT IS OVER THEIR HEAD, NECK OR CHEST.**

TREATMENT FOR A CASUALTY WHO HAS BEEN CRUSHED FOR LESS THAN 15 MINUTES

- If it's possible, release the casualty from the crush as soon as you can
- Remember your first aid priorities and treat appropriately:
  - Breathing
  - Bleeding (takes priority over their airway if it is catastrophic)
  - Burns and breaks
- Treat for shock and call for an ambulance

TREATMENT FOR A CASUALTY WHO HAS BEEN CRUSHED FOR MORE THAN 15 MINUTES

- Do not remove the item that is crushing your casualty
- Call for an ambulance
- Monitor their response levels continuously
- Offer them plenty of reassurance
- Treat them for shock

If you are in a remote setting and professional help is not available, consider applying a tourniquet above the injured area before lifting the crushing object, if it is safe and you are trained to do so.

HYPOTHERMIA

Hypothermia occurs when a person's normal body temperature of around 37°C (98.6°F) drops below 35°C (95°F). It is usually caused by being in a cold environment. It can be triggered by a combination of things, including prolonged exposure to cold (such as staying outdoors in cold conditions for a long period of time), rain, wind, sweat, inactivity or being in cold water.

The casualty's age and general health condition plays a large part in the development of hypothermia as well as medical conditions, such as circulatory illness (shock, heart attack) or injury to the head and spine.

Signs and symptoms

The symptoms of hypothermia depend on how cold the environment is and how long your casualty is exposed for. Severe hypothermia needs urgent medical treatment in hospital. Shivering is a good guide to how severe the condition is. If the person can stop shivering on their own, the hypothermia is mild, but if they cannot stop shivering, it could be moderate to severe.

NB: If the casualty is not shivering, it could be that the casualty is in a severe hypothermic state.

Mild cases	Moderate cases	Severe cases
Shivering	Violent, uncontrollable shivering	Loss of control of hands, feet and limbs
Feeling cold	Being unable to think straight or pay attention	Uncontrollable shivering that suddenly stops
Low energy	Confusion (some people don't realise they are affected)	Shallow or no breathing
Cold, pale skin	Loss of judgement and reasoning	Weak, irregular or no pulse
	Difficulty moving around or stumbling (weakness)	Stiff muscles
	Feeling afraid	Dilated pupils
	Memory loss	Unresponsiveness
	Fumbling hands and loss of coordination	
	Drowsiness	
	Slurred speech	
	Slow, shallow breathing and a weak pulse	

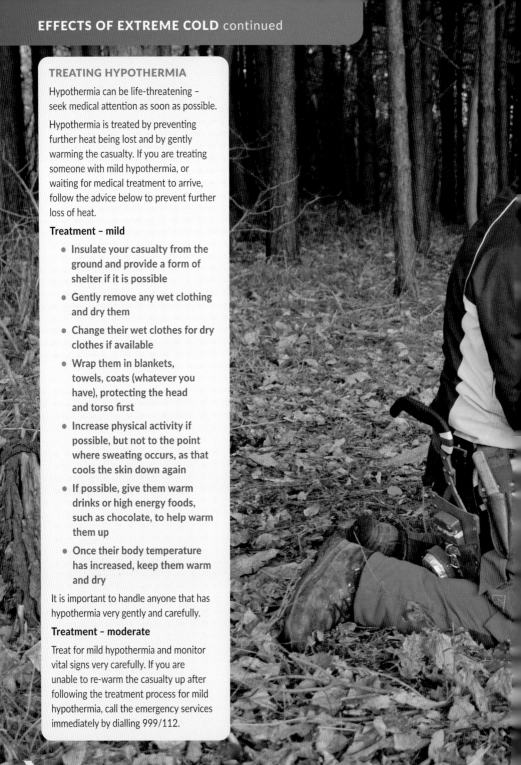

TREATING HYPOTHERMIA

Hypothermia can be life-threatening – seek medical attention as soon as possible.

Hypothermia is treated by preventing further heat being lost and by gently warming the casualty. If you are treating someone with mild hypothermia, or waiting for medical treatment to arrive, follow the advice below to prevent further loss of heat.

Treatment – mild

- Insulate your casualty from the ground and provide a form of shelter if it is possible
- Gently remove any wet clothing and dry them
- Change their wet clothes for dry clothes if available
- Wrap them in blankets, towels, coats (whatever you have), protecting the head and torso first
- Increase physical activity if possible, but not to the point where sweating occurs, as that cools the skin down again
- If possible, give them warm drinks or high energy foods, such as chocolate, to help warm them up
- Once their body temperature has increased, keep them warm and dry

It is important to handle anyone that has hypothermia very gently and carefully.

Treatment – moderate

Treat for mild hypothermia and monitor vital signs very carefully. If you are unable to re-warm the casualty up after following the treatment process for mild hypothermia, call the emergency services immediately by dialling 999/112.

Cases of severe hypothermia require urgent medical treatment in hospital. You should call for professional medical assistance if you suspect your casualty has a case of severe hypothermia.

Treatment – severe

- **Handle your casualty very gently and carefully**
- **Provide shelter and insulate your casualty from the ground**
- **Place them into the recovery position and monitor vital signs**

Do not give them any food or drink. As the body temperature drops, shivering will stop completely. The heart rate will slow and your casualty will gradually lose responsiveness. Be prepared to resuscitate if they stop breathing normally.

THINGS YOU SHOULD **NOT DO**

Do not apply direct heat (hot water or a heating pad, for example) to the arms and legs, as this forces cold blood back to the major organs, making the condition worse.

Do not give them alcohol to drink, as this will decrease the body's ability to retain heat.

Do not rub or massage their skin, as this can cause the blood vessels to widen and decrease the body's ability to retain heat. In severe cases of hypothermia there is also a risk of a heart attack.

LYME DISEASE

TICKS

Ticks are tiny, eight-legged creatures that survive by feeding on the blood of animals and humans. Technically speaking, ticks are not insects, they fall into the same category as spiders - Arachnids.

Ticks can be found in areas with thick vegetation, woodland and moorland areas across the UK and because of their tiny size, they can easily go unnoticed, even after they have bitten you. Ticks are capable of transmitting infections such as Lyme disease, which, if left untreated, can cause severe, long term health problems.

Ticks can attach themselves anywhere on the human body, but mainly warm, moist areas such as the armpit or groin are targeted. Once a tick has found its way onto the body it will bite into the skin and begin to feed. If the tick is not removed properly, the head and mouth parts can remain embedded and become infected.

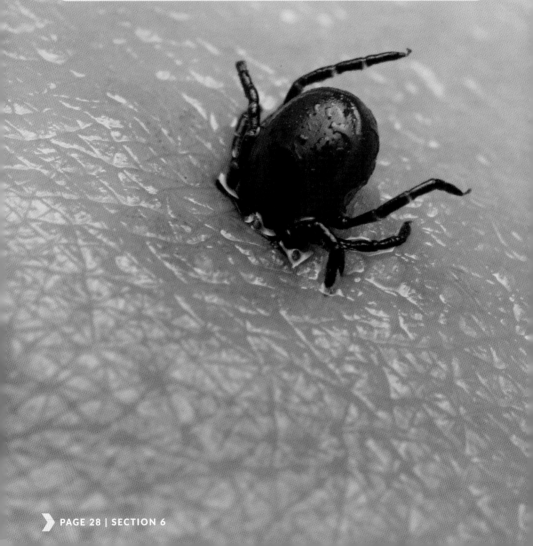

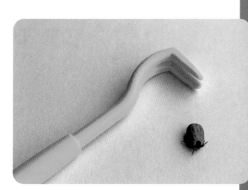

TREATMENT FOR TICK BITES

Remove the tick as soon as possible!

Tick removal tool:

- Wear disposable gloves
- Engage the tool by approaching the tick from the side until it is held securely
- Carefully turn the tool (clockwise or counter-clockwise). The tick should detach itself after 2-3 rotations
- After removing the tick, disinfect the bite site and wash your hands with soap and water

DO NOT rotate or turn the tick using a tick removal tool, unless the manufacturer's instructions tell you to do so.

Fine-tipped tweezers:

- Wear disposable gloves
- Gently grip the tick using fine-tipped tweezers, getting as close to the skin as possible
- Pull upwards very slowly and carefully without crushing the tick. If the head and mouth parts remain, the body will be susceptible to infection
- Once you have successfully removed the tick, wash your skin with clean water
- Apply an antiseptic cream to the skin around the bite
- Keep an eye on the bitten area for several weeks afterwards and if you begin to feel unwell, visit your GP

LYME DISEASE

Lyme disease is an infectious disease which can be carried by ticks. In the majority of cases, the disease is transmitted to humans by infected ticks biting and feeding on the blood.

Once the tick has bitten into the skin, it will attach itself very firmly and begin feeding on the blood. Bacteria from an infected tick can enter our blood stream which can lead to infections including Lyme disease.

Lyme disease can affect any part of the body and can cause a variety of symptoms, including:

Early stages	Later stages
Tiredness and fatigue	More serious symptoms may develop several weeks, months or even years later if left untreated.
Nausea	
Muscle and joint pain	Distinctive circular rash (may appear 3-30 days after being bitten)
Headache	
High temperature	Pain and swelling in the joints
Chills	Numbness and pain in the limbs
Neck stiffness	Paralysis of facial muscles
	Memory problems
	Heart problems

If any of the above symptoms develop after being bitten by a tick, or if you think you have been bitten, visit your GP.

TICK BITE PREVENTION

- Wear trousers as opposed to shorts
- Tuck clothes in, such as trousers into socks
- Wear light coloured clothing rather Than dark
- Try to stay on footpaths and avoid walking through long grass
- Brush off your clothing after walking through areas of vegetation
- Consider using an insect repellent (products containing DEET are best)
- Check yourself over at the end of each working day

WHAT IS SUSPENSION TRAUMA?

Suspension trauma *(also known as suspension syncope, harness hang syndrome or orthostatic intolerance)* occurs when a person is left suspended upright in a safety harness without any physical movement for a period of time.

Being held in this position for a prolonged period of time significantly increases the risk of oxygen deprivation which, if left untreated, can cause severe brain damage and ultimately, death.

When personal fall protection systems are used to work at height, it is imperative that a rescue plan has been implemented to ensure the health and safety of those utilising the equipment.

Depending on the scale of the work and the risks involved, the local emergency service departments should be informed so that they can anticipate a rescue at height during the time frame provided.

When someone falls from height and is left suspended vertically, prompt rescue is very important to ensure they do not suffer from the effects of suspension trauma.

Syncope

Syncope is a temporary loss of consciousness due to insufficient blood flow to the brain *(commonly known as fainting)*. When a person almost, but doesn't actually lose consciousness, is known as presyncope.

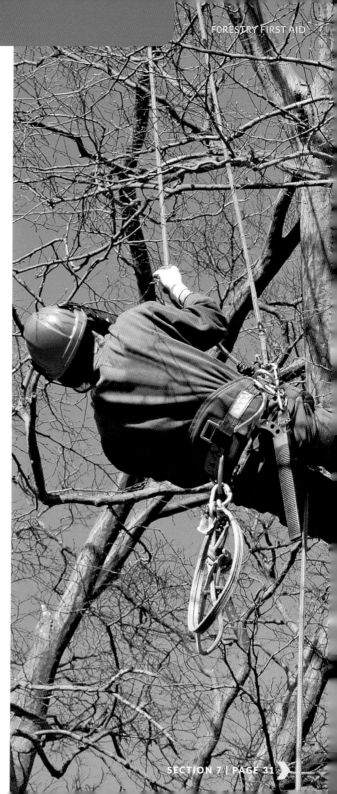

Figure 1 - The Mechanism of Suspension Trauma

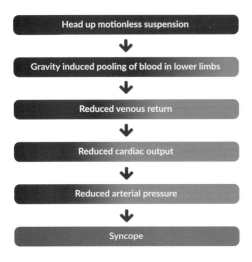

Head up motionless suspension
↓
Gravity induced pooling of blood in lower limbs
↓
Reduced venous return
↓
Reduced cardiac output
↓
Reduced arterial pressure
↓
Syncope

SIGNS AND SYMPTOMS

The early symptoms of suspension trauma can occur in a matter of minutes:

- Light-headedness
- Nausea
- Sensations of flushing
- Tingling or numbness of the arms or legs
- Anxiety
- Visual disturbance
- Pallor
- Feeling as though they are about to faint

If the person remains suspended without any physical interventions, syncope will consequentially follow. Symptoms may appear in 1 in 5 casualty's within 10 minutes *(but generally after being suspended for 60 minutes or longer).*

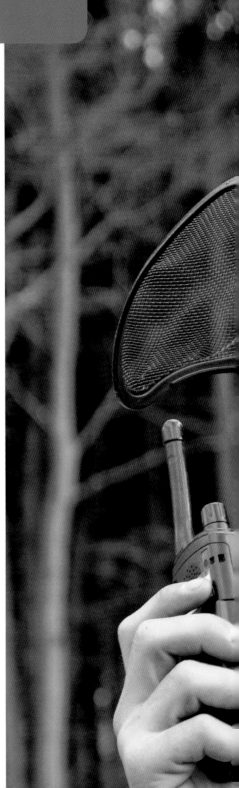

TREATMENT

A rescue plan is a critical part of your fall protection arrangements. A casualty who is experiencing pre-syncopal symptoms, or who is unresponsive whilst suspended in a harness, should be rescued as soon as it's safe to do so.

Your role as a First Aider includes recognising the signs and symptoms, contacting the emergency services and administering first aid following the basic life support protocol.

- If you are unable to immediately release the casualty from the suspended position, elevation of the legs by the casualty themselves or by rescuers may prolong tolerance of suspension
- Keep talking to the casualty and provide reassurance
- Consider removing the person from suspension in the direction of gravity i.e. downwards if you are trained to do so and it does not delay the rescue
- Following rescue, carry out your basic life support procedures (DR ABC)
- If they become unresponsive, call 999 for an ambulance

FURTHER READING:

Health and Safety Executive (HSE) RR708 Research Report 2009

Evidence-based review of the current guidance on first aid measures for suspension trauma

LIGHTNING STRIKE AND HIGH-VOLTAGE INJURIES

Injuries from lightning strikes or high-voltage electrical supplies (e.g. overhead power lines) can be life-threatening.

You may have multiple injuries to treat, including cessation of breathing, and a wound that enters the body as well as one that exits the body. Your first priority is to ensure that it is safe to offer your casualty treatment.

In respect of a high-voltage electrical injury, it is imperative that you and all bystanders stay well away from your casualty. Because the supply can 'arc', you must stay at least 18 metres away from the supply source.

You must call the emergency services immediately, detailing the extent of the incident. As soon as you have deemed it safe to do so, you may start your treatment.

Signs and symptoms:

- **Severe thermal burns**
- **Entry and exit burns, particularly with lightning strikes**
- **Breathing difficulties**
- **Heart palpitations**
- **Muscle, nerve and tissue damage**
- **Dizziness and confusion**
- **Seizure**
- **Loss of responsiveness**
- **Cardiac arrest**

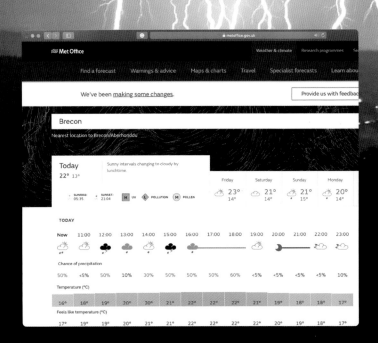

TREATMENTS

Lightning strike injuries

Only when it is safe to do so:

- Carry out your basic life support procedures
- Call the emergency services
- Be aware of any potential serious burns to deal with

High-voltage electrical injuries

Keep everyone at least 18 metres away from the electrical source

- Call the emergency services
- Do not touch the casualty if they are still in contact with the electrical current
- Only when it is safe to do so, as directed by the emergency services, carry out your basic life support procedures

SAFETY TIPS FOR WHEN LIGHTNING STRIKES

Check the weather conditions in advance and avoid working outside during thundery conditions.

- If it is safe for you to do so, descend to lower ground
- Seek shelter inside a building or vehicle if it is possible
- Avoid sheltering beneath tall, isolated trees or wide, open spaces
- Place any electrical items or metal objects away from your body
- Insulate yourself from the ground by sitting on a rucksack and lifting your feet off the ground
- If you have nowhere to shelter and you cannot insulate yourself from the ground, make yourself as small as possible by crouching down with your feet together, hands on knees and your head tucked in until the storm calms
- Do not seek refuge in close proximity to a watercourse or any form of standing water

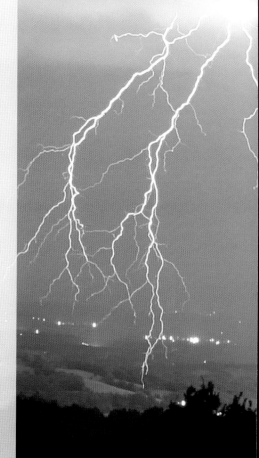

SNAKE BITES

Snakes sometimes bite in self-defence if they are disturbed or provoked. Adders (or vipers) are the only wild venomous snakes in the UK.

Adders sometimes bite without injecting venom (toxins produced by the snake). This is called a 'dry' bite and may cause:

- Mild pain caused by the adder's teeth puncturing the skin
- Anxiety

If an adder injects venom when it bites, it can cause more serious symptoms including:

- Severe pain
- Breathing difficulties
- Swelling and redness in the area of the bite
- Vomiting and diarrhoea
- Mental confusion, dizziness or fainting
- Itchy lumps on the skin (hives or nettle rash)

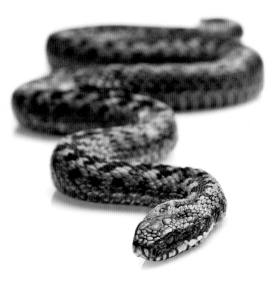

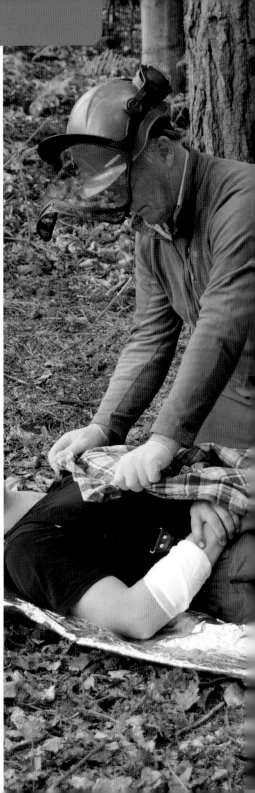